THIS BOOK BELONGS TO:

_____

_____

_____

Health Record Keeper & Journal / A Personal Medical Logbook © 2019 By RealMe Journals
All rights reserved. No part of this book may be used or reproduced in any manner whatsover
without written permissions except in the case of brief quotations embodied in critical articles and reviews.
First Edition: 2019

PERSONAL INFORMATION

Name: _____

Address: _____ City: _____

State/Zip: _____ Home Ph #: _____

Work Ph #: _____ Cell Ph # _____

EMERGENCY CONTACTS

Name: _____

Address: _____ City: _____

State/Zip: _____ Home Ph #: _____

Work Ph #: _____ Cell Ph # _____

Relationship: _____

Name: _____

Address: _____ City: _____

State/Zip: _____ Home Ph #: _____

Work Ph #: _____ Cell Ph # _____

Relationship: _____

Name: _____

Address: _____ City: _____

State/Zip: _____ Home Ph #: _____

Work Ph #: _____ Cell Ph # _____

Relationship: _____

INSURANCE & PHARMACY

Insurance Company: _____

Plan Type: _____ Policyholder: _____

Group #: _____ ID #: _____

Phone #: _____ Website: _____

Username: _____ Password: _____

Insurance Company: _____

Plan Type: _____ Policyholder: _____

Group #: _____ ID #: _____

Phone #: _____ Website: _____

Username: _____ Password: _____

Insurance Company: _____

Plan Type: _____ Policyholder: _____

Group #: _____ ID #: _____

Phone #: _____ Website: _____

Username: _____ Password: _____

PHARMACY INFORMATION

Name:	Name:
Phone:	Phone:
Fax:	Fax:
Location:	Location:

FAMILY MEDICAL HISTORY

LIST FAMILY MEMBER IN TOP ROW

MEDICAL CONDITION				
High Blood Pressure				
Diabetes				
High Cholesterol				
Heart Disease				
Stroke/TIA				
Allergies				
Auto Immune Diseases				
Cancer				
Arthritis				
Birth Defects				
Infertility				
Mental Illness				
Kidney Disease				
Liver Disease				
Lung Disease				
Blood Disorder				
Gastrointestinal Disorder				
Nerve Disorders				
Migraines				
Endometriosis				

FAMILY MEDICAL HISTORY

LIST FAMILY MEMBER IN TOP ROW

			NOTES

FAMILY MEDICAL HISTORY

LIST FAMILY MEMBER IN TOP ROW

MEDICAL CONDITION					

FAMILY MEDICAL HISTORY

LIST FAMILY MEMBER IN TOP ROW

			NOTES

MY MEDICAL QUICK VIEW

Name: _____ Donor: Y / N _____

Date of Birth: _____ Blood Type: _____

Height: _____ Weight: _____

MEDICAL CONDITIONS

- High Blood Pressure   YES / NO   MEDS: _____
- Diabetic   YES / NO   Insulin / Oral Meds / Both _____
- _____
- _____
- _____
- _____
- _____
- _____
- _____
- _____

ALLERGIES	REACTION	MEDICATION

IMMUNIZATION CHART

VACCINATION	FACILITY	DATE GIVEN	AGE GIVEN	SITE GIVEN

NOTES

NOTES

MEDICATIONS

Medication	Condition	Dose	Frequency	Start Date	End Date

Physician: Notes:

Physician: Notes:

Physician: Notes:

Physician: Notes:

Physician: Notes:

Physician: Notes:

Physician: Notes:

Physician: Notes:

Physician: Notes:

MEDICATIONS

Medication	Condition	Dose	Frequency	Start Date	End Date
Physician:		Notes:			
Physician:		Notes:			
Physician:		Notes:			
Physician:		Notes:			
Physician:		Notes:			
Physician:		Notes:			
Physician:		Notes:			
Physician:		Notes:			
Physician:		Notes:			
Physician:		Notes:			

MEDICATIONS

Medication	Condition	Dose	Frequency	Start Date	End Date
Physician:		Notes:			
Physician:		Notes:			
Physician:		Notes:			
Physician:		Notes:			
Physician:		Notes:			
Physician:		Notes:			
Physician:		Notes:			
Physician:		Notes:			
Physician:		Notes:			
Physician:		Notes:			

MEDICATIONS

Medication	Condition	Dose	Frequency	Start Date	End Date
Physician:		Notes:			
Physician:		Notes:			
Physician:		Notes:			
Physician:		Notes:			
Physician:		Notes:			
Physician:		Notes:			
Physician:		Notes:			
Physician:		Notes:			
Physician:		Notes:			
Physician:		Notes:			

MEDICATIONS

Medication	Condition	Dose	Frequency	Start Date	End Date
Physician:		Notes:			
Physician:		Notes:			
Physician:		Notes:			
Physician:		Notes:			
Physician:		Notes:			
Physician:		Notes:			
Physician:		Notes:			
Physician:		Notes:			
Physician:		Notes:			
Physician:		Notes:			

MEDICATIONS

Medication	Condition	Dose	Frequency	Start Date	End Date

Physician: Notes:

Physician: Notes:

Physician: Notes:

Physician: Notes:

Physician: Notes:

Physician: Notes:

Physician: Notes:

Physician: Notes:

Physician: Notes:

MY PHYSICIANS

PRIMARY CARE DOCTOR

Name: _____

Address: _____

Phone: _____

Patient Portal Website: _____

Username: _____ Password: _____

OB/GYN

Name: _____

Address: _____

Phone: _____

Patient Portal Website: _____

Username: _____ Password: _____

EYE DOCTOR

Name: _____

Address: _____

Phone: _____

Patient Portal Website: _____

Username: _____ Password: _____

MY PHYSICIANS

PRIMARY CARE DOCTOR

Name:

Address:

Phone:

Patient Portal Website:

Username: Password:

OB/GYN

Name:

Address:

Phone:

Patient Portal Website:

Username: Password:

EYE DOCTOR

Name:

Address:

Phone:

Patient Portal Website:

Username: Password:

MY PHYSICIANS

PRIMARY CARE DOCTOR

Name: _____

Address: _____

Phone: _____

Patient Portal Website: _____

Username: _____ Password: _____

OB/GYN

Name: _____

Address: _____

Phone: _____

Patient Portal Website: _____

Username: _____ Password: _____

EYE DOCTOR

Name: _____

Address: _____

Phone: _____

Patient Portal Website: _____

Username: _____ Password: _____

HOSPITAL & RADIOLOGY

HOSPITAL #1

Name:

Address:

Phone:

Patient Portal Website:

Username: Password:

HOSPITAL #2

Name:

Address:

Phone:

Patient Portal Website:

Username: Password:

IMAGING CENTER

Name:

Address:

Phone:

Patient Portal Website:

Username: Password:

SURGICAL HISTORY

Procedure:	Date:
Hospital:	Physician:

☐ Right ☐ Left ☐ Both ☐ N/A

NOTES:

Procedure:	Date:
Hospital:	Physician:

☐ Right ☐ Left ☐ Both ☐ N/A

NOTES:

SURGICAL HISTORY

Procedure:	Date:
Hospital:	Physician:

☐ Right ☐ Left ☐ Both ☐ N/A

NOTES:

Procedure:	Date:
Hospital:	Physician:

☐ Right ☐ Left ☐ Both ☐ N/A

NOTES:

SURGICAL HISTORY

Procedure:	Date:
Hospital:	Physician:

☐ Right ☐ Left ☐ Both ☐ N/A

NOTES:
_____
_____
_____
_____
_____
_____
_____

Procedure:	Date:
Hospital:	Physician:

☐ Right ☐ Left ☐ Both ☐ N/A

NOTES:
_____
_____
_____
_____
_____
_____
_____

SURGICAL HISTORY

Procedure:	Date:
Hospital:	Physician:

☐ Right ☐ Left ☐ Both ☐ N/A

NOTES:

Procedure:	Date:
Hospital:	Physician:

☐ Right ☐ Left ☐ Both ☐ N/A

NOTES:

SURGICAL HISTORY

Procedure:	Date:
Hospital:	Physician:

☐ Right ☐ Left ☐ Both ☐ N/A

NOTES:
\
\
\
\
\
\

Procedure:	Date:
Hospital:	Physician:

☐ Right ☐ Left ☐ Both ☐ N/A

NOTES:
\
\
\
\
\
\

SURGICAL HISTORY

Procedure:	Date:
Hospital:	Physician:

☐ Right ☐ Left ☐ Both ☐ N/A

NOTES:
\
\
\
\
\
\
\

Procedure:	Date:
Hospital:	Physician:

☐ Right ☐ Left ☐ Both ☐ N/A

NOTES:
\
\
\
\
\
\
\

SURGICAL HISTORY

Procedure:	Date:
Hospital:	Physician:

☐ Right ☐ Left ☐ Both ☐ N/A
NOTES:

Procedure:	Date:
Hospital:	Physician:

☐ Right ☐ Left ☐ Both ☐ N/A
NOTES:

SURGICAL HISTORY

Procedure:	Date:
Hospital:	Physician:

☐ Right ☐ Left ☐ Both ☐ N/A

NOTES:
\
\
\
\
\
\
\

Procedure:	Date:
Hospital:	Physician:

☐ Right ☐ Left ☐ Both ☐ N/A

NOTES:
\
\
\
\
\
\
\

NOTES

NOTES

EMERGENCY ROOM/URGENT CARE

Facility/Dr.:	Date:
Reason:	
Tests:	
Results:	
Discharge Instructions:	

Facility/Dr.:	Date:
Reason:	
Tests:	
Results:	
Discharge Instructions:	

Facility/Dr.:	Date:
Reason:	
Tests:	
Results:	
Discharge Instructions:	

EMERGENCY ROOM/URGENT CARE

Facility/Dr.:	Date:
Reason:	
Tests:	
Results:	
Discharge Instructions:	

Facility/Dr.:	Date:
Reason:	
Tests:	
Results:	
Discharge Instructions:	

Facility/Dr.:	Date:
Reason:	
Tests:	
Results:	
Discharge Instructions:	

EMERGENCY ROOM/URGENT CARE

Facility/Dr.:	Date:
Reason:	
Tests:	
Results:	
Discharge Instructions:	

Facility/Dr.:	Date:
Reason:	
Tests:	
Results:	
Discharge Instructions:	

Facility/Dr.:	Date:
Reason:	
Tests:	
Results:	
Discharge Instructions:	

EMERGENCY ROOM/URGENT CARE

Facility/Dr.:	Date:

Reason:

Tests:

Results:

Discharge Instructions:

Facility/Dr.:	Date:

Reason:

Tests:

Results:

Discharge Instructions:

Facility/Dr.:	Date:

Reason:

Tests:

Results:

Discharge Instructions:

EMERGENCY ROOM/URGENT CARE

Facility/Dr.:	Date:
Reason:	
Tests:	
Results:	
Discharge Instructions:	

Facility/Dr.:	Date:
Reason:	
Tests:	
Results:	
Discharge Instructions:	

Facility/Dr.:	Date:
Reason:	
Tests:	
Results:	
Discharge Instructions:	

EMERGENCY ROOM/URGENT CARE

Facility/Dr.:	Date:
Reason:	
Tests:	
Results:	
Discharge Instructions:	

Facility/Dr.:	Date:
Reason:	
Tests:	
Results:	
Discharge Instructions:	

Facility/Dr.:	Date:
Reason:	
Tests:	
Results:	
Discharge Instructions:	

EMERGENCY ROOM/URGENT CARE

Facility/Dr.:	Date:

Reason:

Tests:

Results:

Discharge Instructions:

Facility/Dr.:	Date:

Reason:

Tests:

Results:

Discharge Instructions:

Facility/Dr.:	Date:

Reason:

Tests:

Results:

Discharge Instructions:

EMERGENCY ROOM/URGENT CARE

Facility/Dr.:	Date:

Reason:

Tests:

Results:

Discharge Instructions:

Facility/Dr.:	Date:

Reason:

Tests:

Results:

Discharge Instructions:

Facility/Dr.:	Date:

Reason:

Tests:

Results:

Discharge Instructions:

EMERGENCY ROOM/URGENT CARE

Facility/Dr.:	Date:
Reason:	
Tests:	
Results:	
Discharge Instructions:	

Facility/Dr.:	Date:
Reason:	
Tests:	
Results:	
Discharge Instructions:	

Facility/Dr.:	Date:
Reason:	
Tests:	
Results:	
Discharge Instructions:	

EMERGENCY ROOM/URGENT CARE

Facility/Dr.:	Date:
Reason:	
Tests:	
Results:	
Discharge Instructions:	

Facility/Dr.:	Date:
Reason:	
Tests:	
Results:	
Discharge Instructions:	

Facility/Dr.:	Date:
Reason:	
Tests:	
Results:	
Discharge Instructions:	

NOTES

NOTES

DOCTOR VISITS

Date:	Appt Time:
Physician:	Specialty:
Reason For Visit:	

QUESTIONS/CONCERNS

VITALS

Height:	Weight:
Blood Pressure:	Pulse Rate:
Blood Glucose:	Temperature:

MEDICATION UPDATES

Medication	Dosage	Frequency	Duration

PHYSICIAN DIAGNOSIS / DISCUSSION

TESTS ORDERED

Test/Exam:	Facility
Date:	Appt time:
Prep For Test:	
Test Results:	

Test/Exam:	Facility
Date:	Appt time:
Prep For Test:	
Test Results:	

Test/Exam:	Facility
Date:	Appt time:
Prep For Test:	
Test Results:	

DOCTOR VISITS

Date:	Appt Time:
Physician:	Specialty:
Reason For Visit:	

QUESTIONS/CONCERNS

VITALS

Height:	Weight:
Blood Pressure:	Pulse Rate:
Blood Glucose:	Temperature:

MEDICATION UPDATES

Medication	Dosage	Frequency	Duration

PHYSICIAN DIAGNOSIS / DISCUSSION

TESTS ORDERED

Test/Exam:	Facility
Date:	Appt time:
Prep For Test:	
Test Results:	

Test/Exam:	Facility
Date:	Appt time:
Prep For Test:	
Test Results:	

Test/Exam:	Facility
Date:	Appt time:
Prep For Test:	
Test Results:	

DOCTOR VISITS

Date:	Appt Time:
Physician:	Specialty:
Reason For Visit:	

QUESTIONS/CONCERNS

VITALS

Height:	Weight:
Blood Pressure:	Pulse Rate:
Blood Glucose:	Temperature:

MEDICATION UPDATES

Medication	Dosage	Frequency	Duration

PHYSICIAN DIAGNOSIS / DISCUSSION

TESTS ORDERED

Test/Exam:	Facility
Date:	Appt time:
Prep For Test:	
Test Results:	

Test/Exam:	Facility
Date:	Appt time:
Prep For Test:	
Test Results:	

Test/Exam:	Facility
Date:	Appt time:
Prep For Test:	
Test Results:	

DOCTOR VISITS

Date:	Appt Time:
Physician:	Specialty:
Reason For Visit:	

QUESTIONS/CONCERNS

VITALS

Height:	Weight:
Blood Pressure:	Pulse Rate:
Blood Glucose:	Temperature:

MEDICATION UPDATES

Medication	Dosage	Frequency	Duration

PHYSICIAN DIAGNOSIS / DISCUSSION

TESTS ORDERED

Test/Exam:	Facility
Date:	Appt time:
Prep For Test:	
Test Results:	

Test/Exam:	Facility
Date:	Appt time:
Prep For Test:	
Test Results:	

Test/Exam:	Facility
Date:	Appt time:
Prep For Test:	
Test Results:	

DOCTOR VISITS

Date:	Appt Time:
Physician:	Specialty:
Reason For Visit:	

QUESTIONS/CONCERNS

VITALS

Height:	Weight:
Blood Pressure:	Pulse Rate:
Blood Glucose:	Temperature:

MEDICATION UPDATES

Medication	Dosage	Frequency	Duration

PHYSICIAN DIAGNOSIS / DISCUSSION

TESTS ORDERED

Test/Exam:	Facility
Date:	Appt time:
Prep For Test:	
Test Results:	

Test/Exam:	Facility
Date:	Appt time:
Prep For Test:	
Test Results:	

Test/Exam:	Facility
Date:	Appt time:
Prep For Test:	
Test Results:	

DOCTOR VISITS

Date:	Appt Time:
Physician:	Specialty:
Reason For Visit:	

QUESTIONS/CONCERNS

VITALS

Height:	Weight:
Blood Pressure:	Pulse Rate:
Blood Glucose:	Temperature:

MEDICATION UPDATES

Medication	Dosage	Frequency	Duration

PHYSICIAN DIAGNOSIS / DISCUSSION

TESTS ORDERED

Test/Exam:	Facility
Date:	Appt time:
Prep For Test:	
Test Results:	

Test/Exam:	Facility
Date:	Appt time:
Prep For Test:	
Test Results:	

Test/Exam:	Facility
Date:	Appt time:
Prep For Test:	
Test Results:	

DOCTOR VISITS

Date:	Appt Time:
Physician:	Specialty:
Reason For Visit:	

QUESTIONS/CONCERNS

VITALS

Height:	Weight:
Blood Pressure:	Pulse Rate:
Blood Glucose:	Temperature:

MEDICATION UPDATES

Medication	Dosage	Frequency	Duration

PHYSICIAN DIAGNOSIS / DISCUSSION

TESTS ORDERED

Test/Exam:	Facility
Date:	Appt time:
Prep For Test:	
Test Results:	

Test/Exam:	Facility
Date:	Appt time:
Prep For Test:	
Test Results:	

Test/Exam:	Facility
Date:	Appt time:
Prep For Test:	
Test Results:	

DOCTOR VISITS

Date:	Appt Time:
Physician:	Specialty:
Reason For Visit:	

QUESTIONS/CONCERNS

VITALS

Height:	Weight:
Blood Pressure:	Pulse Rate:
Blood Glucose:	Temperature:

MEDICATION UPDATES

Medication	Dosage	Frequency	Duration

PHYSICIAN DIAGNOSIS / DISCUSSION

TESTS ORDERED

Test/Exam:	Facility
Date:	Appt time:
Prep For Test:	
Test Results:	

Test/Exam:	Facility
Date:	Appt time:
Prep For Test:	
Test Results:	

Test/Exam:	Facility
Date:	Appt time:
Prep For Test:	
Test Results:	

DOCTOR VISITS

Date:	Appt Time:
Physician:	Specialty:
Reason For Visit:	

QUESTIONS/CONCERNS

VITALS

Height:	Weight:
Blood Pressure:	Pulse Rate:
Blood Glucose:	Temperature:

MEDICATION UPDATES

Medication	Dosage	Frequency	Duration

PHYSICIAN DIAGNOSIS / DISCUSSION

TESTS ORDERED

Test/Exam:	Facility
Date:	Appt time:
Prep For Test:	
Test Results:	

Test/Exam:	Facility
Date:	Appt time:
Prep For Test:	
Test Results:	

Test/Exam:	Facility
Date:	Appt time:
Prep For Test:	
Test Results:	

DOCTOR VISITS

Date:	Appt Time:
Physician:	Specialty:
Reason For Visit:	

QUESTIONS/CONCERNS

VITALS

Height:	Weight:
Blood Pressure:	Pulse Rate:
Blood Glucose:	Temperature:

MEDICATION UPDATES

Medication	Dosage	Frequency	Duration

PHYSICIAN DIAGNOSIS / DISCUSSION

TESTS ORDERED

Test/Exam:	Facility
Date:	Appt time:
Prep For Test:	
Test Results:	

Test/Exam:	Facility
Date:	Appt time:
Prep For Test:	
Test Results:	

Test/Exam:	Facility
Date:	Appt time:
Prep For Test:	
Test Results:	

DOCTOR VISITS

Date:	Appt Time:
Physician:	Specialty:
Reason For Visit:	

QUESTIONS/CONCERNS

VITALS

Height:	Weight:
Blood Pressure:	Pulse Rate:
Blood Glucose:	Temperature:

MEDICATION UPDATES

Medication	Dosage	Frequency	Duration

PHYSICIAN DIAGNOSIS / DISCUSSION

TESTS ORDERED

Test/Exam:	Facility
Date:	Appt time:
Prep For Test:	
Test Results:	

Test/Exam:	Facility
Date:	Appt time:
Prep For Test:	
Test Results:	

Test/Exam:	Facility
Date:	Appt time:
Prep For Test:	
Test Results:	

DOCTOR VISITS

Date:	Appt Time:
Physician:	Specialty:
Reason For Visit:	

QUESTIONS/CONCERNS

VITALS

Height:	Weight:
Blood Pressure:	Pulse Rate:
Blood Glucose:	Temperature:

MEDICATION UPDATES

Medication	Dosage	Frequency	Duration

PHYSICIAN DIAGNOSIS / DISCUSSION

TESTS ORDERED

Test/Exam:	Facility
Date:	Appt time:
Prep For Test:	
Test Results:	

Test/Exam:	Facility
Date:	Appt time:
Prep For Test:	
Test Results:	

Test/Exam:	Facility
Date:	Appt time:
Prep For Test:	
Test Results:	

DOCTOR VISITS

Date:	Appt Time:
Physician:	Specialty:
Reason For Visit:	

QUESTIONS/CONCERNS

VITALS

Height:	Weight:
Blood Pressure:	Pulse Rate:
Blood Glucose:	Temperature:

MEDICATION UPDATES

Medication	Dosage	Frequency	Duration

PHYSICIAN DIAGNOSIS / DISCUSSION

TESTS ORDERED

Test/Exam:	Facility
Date:	Appt time:
Prep For Test:	
Test Results:	

Test/Exam:	Facility
Date:	Appt time:
Prep For Test:	
Test Results:	

Test/Exam:	Facility
Date:	Appt time:
Prep For Test:	
Test Results:	

DOCTOR VISITS

Date:	Appt Time:
Physician:	Specialty:
Reason For Visit:	

QUESTIONS/CONCERNS

VITALS

Height:	Weight:
Blood Pressure:	Pulse Rate:
Blood Glucose:	Temperature:

MEDICATION UPDATES

Medication	Dosage	Frequency	Duration

PHYSICIAN DIAGNOSIS / DISCUSSION

TESTS ORDERED

Test/Exam:	Facility
Date:	Appt time:
Prep For Test:	
Test Results:	

Test/Exam:	Facility
Date:	Appt time:
Prep For Test:	
Test Results:	

Test/Exam:	Facility
Date:	Appt time:
Prep For Test:	
Test Results:	

DOCTOR VISITS

Date:	Appt Time:
Physician:	Specialty:
Reason For Visit:	

QUESTIONS/CONCERNS

VITALS

Height:	Weight:
Blood Pressure:	Pulse Rate:
Blood Glucose:	Temperature:

MEDICATION UPDATES

Medication	Dosage	Frequency	Duration

PHYSICIAN DIAGNOSIS / DISCUSSION

TESTS ORDERED

Test/Exam:	Facility
Date:	Appt time:
Prep For Test:	
Test Results:	

Test/Exam:	Facility
Date:	Appt time:
Prep For Test:	
Test Results:	

Test/Exam:	Facility
Date:	Appt time:
Prep For Test:	
Test Results:	

DOCTOR VISITS

Date:	Appt Time:
Physician:	Specialty:
Reason For Visit:	

QUESTIONS/CONCERNS

VITALS

Height:	Weight:
Blood Pressure:	Pulse Rate:
Blood Glucose:	Temperature:

MEDICATION UPDATES

Medication	Dosage	Frequency	Duration

PHYSICIAN DIAGNOSIS / DISCUSSION

TESTS ORDERED

Test/Exam:	Facility
Date:	Appt time:
Prep For Test:	
Test Results:	

Test/Exam:	Facility
Date:	Appt time:
Prep For Test:	
Test Results:	

Test/Exam:	Facility
Date:	Appt time:
Prep For Test:	
Test Results:	

DOCTOR VISITS

Date:	Appt Time:
Physician:	Specialty:
Reason For Visit:	

QUESTIONS/CONCERNS

VITALS

Height:	Weight:
Blood Pressure:	Pulse Rate:
Blood Glucose:	Temperature:

MEDICATION UPDATES

Medication	Dosage	Frequency	Duration

PHYSICIAN DIAGNOSIS / DISCUSSION

TESTS ORDERED

Test/Exam:	Facility
Date:	Appt time:
Prep For Test:	
Test Results:	

Test/Exam:	Facility
Date:	Appt time:
Prep For Test:	
Test Results:	

Test/Exam:	Facility
Date:	Appt time:
Prep For Test:	
Test Results:	

DOCTOR VISITS

Date:	Appt Time:
Physician:	Specialty:
Reason For Visit:	

QUESTIONS/CONCERNS

VITALS

Height:	Weight:
Blood Pressure:	Pulse Rate:
Blood Glucose:	Temperature:

MEDICATION UPDATES

Medication	Dosage	Frequency	Duration

PHYSICIAN DIAGNOSIS / DISCUSSION

TESTS ORDERED

Test/Exam:	Facility
Date:	Appt time:
Prep For Test:	
Test Results:	

Test/Exam:	Facility
Date:	Appt time:
Prep For Test:	
Test Results:	

Test/Exam:	Facility
Date:	Appt time:
Prep For Test:	
Test Results:	

DOCTOR VISITS

Date:	Appt Time:
Physician:	Specialty:
Reason For Visit:	

QUESTIONS/CONCERNS

VITALS

Height:	Weight:
Blood Pressure:	Pulse Rate:
Blood Glucose:	Temperature:

MEDICATION UPDATES

Medication	Dosage	Frequency	Duration

PHYSICIAN DIAGNOSIS / DISCUSSION

TESTS ORDERED

Test/Exam:	Facility
Date:	Appt time:
Prep For Test:	
Test Results:	

Test/Exam:	Facility
Date:	Appt time:
Prep For Test:	
Test Results:	

Test/Exam:	Facility
Date:	Appt time:
Prep For Test:	
Test Results:	

DOCTOR VISITS

Date:	Appt Time:
Physician:	Specialty:
Reason For Visit:	

QUESTIONS/CONCERNS

VITALS

Height:	Weight:
Blood Pressure:	Pulse Rate:
Blood Glucose:	Temperature:

MEDICATION UPDATES

Medication	Dosage	Frequency	Duration

PHYSICIAN DIAGNOSIS / DISCUSSION

TESTS ORDERED

Test/Exam:	Facility
Date:	Appt time:
Prep For Test:	
Test Results:	

Test/Exam:	Facility
Date:	Appt time:
Prep For Test:	
Test Results:	

Test/Exam:	Facility
Date:	Appt time:
Prep For Test:	
Test Results:	

DOCTOR VISITS

Date:	Appt Time:
Physician:	Specialty:
Reason For Visit:	

QUESTIONS/CONCERNS

VITALS

Height:	Weight:
Blood Pressure:	Pulse Rate:
Blood Glucose:	Temperature:

MEDICATION UPDATES

Medication	Dosage	Frequency	Duration

PHYSICIAN DIAGNOSIS / DISCUSSION

TESTS ORDERED

Test/Exam:	Facility
Date:	Appt time:
Prep For Test:	
Test Results:	

Test/Exam:	Facility
Date:	Appt time:
Prep For Test:	
Test Results:	

Test/Exam:	Facility
Date:	Appt time:
Prep For Test:	
Test Results:	

DOCTOR VISITS

Date:	Appt Time:
Physician:	Specialty:
Reason For Visit:	

QUESTIONS/CONCERNS

VITALS

Height:	Weight:
Blood Pressure:	Pulse Rate:
Blood Glucose:	Temperature:

MEDICATION UPDATES

Medication	Dosage	Frequency	Duration

PHYSICIAN DIAGNOSIS / DISCUSSION

TESTS ORDERED

Test/Exam:	Facility
Date:	Appt time:
Prep For Test:	
Test Results:	

Test/Exam:	Facility
Date:	Appt time:
Prep For Test:	
Test Results:	

Test/Exam:	Facility
Date:	Appt time:
Prep For Test:	
Test Results:	

DOCTOR VISITS

Date:	Appt Time:
Physician:	Specialty:
Reason For Visit:	

QUESTIONS/CONCERNS

VITALS

Height:	Weight:
Blood Pressure:	Pulse Rate:
Blood Glucose:	Temperature:

MEDICATION UPDATES

Medication	Dosage	Frequency	Duration

PHYSICIAN DIAGNOSIS / DISCUSSION

TESTS ORDERED

Test/Exam:	Facility
Date:	Appt time:
Prep For Test:	
Test Results:	

Test/Exam:	Facility
Date:	Appt time:
Prep For Test:	
Test Results:	

Test/Exam:	Facility
Date:	Appt time:
Prep For Test:	
Test Results:	

DOCTOR VISITS

Date:	Appt Time:
Physician:	Specialty:
Reason For Visit:	

QUESTIONS/CONCERNS

VITALS

Height:	Weight:
Blood Pressure:	Pulse Rate:
Blood Glucose:	Temperature:

MEDICATION UPDATES

Medication	Dosage	Frequency	Duration

PHYSICIAN DIAGNOSIS / DISCUSSION

TESTS ORDERED

Test/Exam:	Facility
Date:	Appt time:
Prep For Test:	
Test Results:	

Test/Exam:	Facility
Date:	Appt time:
Prep For Test:	
Test Results:	

Test/Exam:	Facility
Date:	Appt time:
Prep For Test:	
Test Results:	

DOCTOR VISITS

Date:	Appt Time:
Physician:	Specialty:
Reason For Visit:	

QUESTIONS/CONCERNS

VITALS

Height:	Weight:
Blood Pressure:	Pulse Rate:
Blood Glucose:	Temperature:

MEDICATION UPDATES

Medication	Dosage	Frequency	Duration

PHYSICIAN DIAGNOSIS / DISCUSSION

TESTS ORDERED

Test/Exam:	Facility
Date:	Appt time:
Prep For Test:	
Test Results:	

Test/Exam:	Facility
Date:	Appt time:
Prep For Test:	
Test Results:	

Test/Exam:	Facility
Date:	Appt time:
Prep For Test:	
Test Results:	

DOCTOR VISITS

Date:	Appt Time:
Physician:	Specialty:
Reason For Visit:	

QUESTIONS/CONCERNS

VITALS

Height:	Weight:
Blood Pressure:	Pulse Rate:
Blood Glucose:	Temperature:

MEDICATION UPDATES

Medication	Dosage	Frequency	Duration

PHYSICIAN DIAGNOSIS / DISCUSSION

TESTS ORDERED

Test/Exam:	Facility
Date:	Appt time:
Prep For Test:	
Test Results:	

Test/Exam:	Facility
Date:	Appt time:
Prep For Test:	
Test Results:	

Test/Exam:	Facility
Date:	Appt time:
Prep For Test:	
Test Results:	

DOCTOR VISITS

Date:	Appt Time:
Physician:	Specialty:
Reason For Visit:	

QUESTIONS/CONCERNS

VITALS

Height:	Weight:
Blood Pressure:	Pulse Rate:
Blood Glucose:	Temperature:

MEDICATION UPDATES

Medication	Dosage	Frequency	Duration

PHYSICIAN DIAGNOSIS / DISCUSSION

TESTS ORDERED

Test/Exam:	Facility
Date:	Appt time:
Prep For Test:	
Test Results:	

Test/Exam:	Facility
Date:	Appt time:
Prep For Test:	
Test Results:	

Test/Exam:	Facility
Date:	Appt time:
Prep For Test:	
Test Results:	

DOCTOR VISITS

Date:	Appt Time:
Physician:	Specialty:
Reason For Visit:	

QUESTIONS/CONCERNS

VITALS

Height:	Weight:
Blood Pressure:	Pulse Rate:
Blood Glucose:	Temperature:

MEDICATION UPDATES

Medication	Dosage	Frequency	Duration

PHYSICIAN DIAGNOSIS / DISCUSSION

TESTS ORDERED

Test/Exam:	Facility
Date:	Appt time:
Prep For Test:	
Test Results:	

Test/Exam:	Facility
Date:	Appt time:
Prep For Test:	
Test Results:	

Test/Exam:	Facility
Date:	Appt time:
Prep For Test:	
Test Results:	

DOCTOR VISITS

Date:	Appt Time:
Physician:	Specialty:
Reason For Visit:	

QUESTIONS/CONCERNS

VITALS

Height:	Weight:
Blood Pressure:	Pulse Rate:
Blood Glucose:	Temperature:

MEDICATION UPDATES

Medication	Dosage	Frequency	Duration

PHYSICIAN DIAGNOSIS / DISCUSSION

TESTS ORDERED

Test/Exam:	Facility
Date:	Appt time:
Prep For Test:	
Test Results:	

Test/Exam:	Facility
Date:	Appt time:
Prep For Test:	
Test Results:	

Test/Exam:	Facility
Date:	Appt time:
Prep For Test:	
Test Results:	

DOCTOR VISITS

Date:	Appt Time:
Physician:	Specialty:
Reason For Visit:	

QUESTIONS/CONCERNS

VITALS

Height:	Weight:
Blood Pressure:	Pulse Rate:
Blood Glucose:	Temperature:

MEDICATION UPDATES

Medication	Dosage	Frequency	Duration

PHYSICIAN DIAGNOSIS / DISCUSSION

TESTS ORDERED

Test/Exam:	Facility
Date:	Appt time:
Prep For Test:	
Test Results:	

Test/Exam:	Facility
Date:	Appt time:
Prep For Test:	
Test Results:	

Test/Exam:	Facility
Date:	Appt time:
Prep For Test:	
Test Results:	

DOCTOR VISITS

Date:	Appt Time:
Physician:	Specialty:
Reason For Visit:	

QUESTIONS/CONCERNS

VITALS

Height:	Weight:
Blood Pressure:	Pulse Rate:
Blood Glucose:	Temperature:

MEDICATION UPDATES

Medication	Dosage	Frequency	Duration

PHYSICIAN DIAGNOSIS / DISCUSSION

TESTS ORDERED

Test/Exam:	Facility
Date:	Appt time:
Prep For Test:	
Test Results:	

Test/Exam:	Facility
Date:	Appt time:
Prep For Test:	
Test Results:	

Test/Exam:	Facility
Date:	Appt time:
Prep For Test:	
Test Results:	

DOCTOR VISITS

Date:	Appt Time:
Physician:	Specialty:
Reason For Visit:	

QUESTIONS/CONCERNS

VITALS

Height:	Weight:
Blood Pressure:	Pulse Rate:
Blood Glucose:	Temperature:

MEDICATION UPDATES

Medication	Dosage	Frequency	Duration

PHYSICIAN DIAGNOSIS / DISCUSSION

TESTS ORDERED

Test/Exam:	Facility
Date:	Appt time:
Prep For Test:	
Test Results:	

Test/Exam:	Facility
Date:	Appt time:
Prep For Test:	
Test Results:	

Test/Exam:	Facility
Date:	Appt time:
Prep For Test:	
Test Results:	

DOCTOR VISITS

Date:	Appt Time:
Physician:	Specialty:
Reason For Visit:	

QUESTIONS/CONCERNS

VITALS

Height:	Weight:
Blood Pressure:	Pulse Rate:
Blood Glucose:	Temperature:

MEDICATION UPDATES

Medication	Dosage	Frequency	Duration

PHYSICIAN DIAGNOSIS / DISCUSSION

TESTS ORDERED

Test/Exam:	Facility
Date:	Appt time:
Prep For Test:	
Test Results:	

Test/Exam:	Facility
Date:	Appt time:
Prep For Test:	
Test Results:	

Test/Exam:	Facility
Date:	Appt time:
Prep For Test:	
Test Results:	

DOCTOR VISITS

Date:	Appt Time:
Physician:	Specialty:
Reason For Visit:	

QUESTIONS/CONCERNS

VITALS

Height:	Weight:
Blood Pressure:	Pulse Rate:
Blood Glucose:	Temperature:

MEDICATION UPDATES

Medication	Dosage	Frequency	Duration

PHYSICIAN DIAGNOSIS / DISCUSSION

TESTS ORDERED

Test/Exam:	Facility
Date:	Appt time:
Prep For Test:	
Test Results:	

Test/Exam:	Facility
Date:	Appt time:
Prep For Test:	
Test Results:	

Test/Exam:	Facility
Date:	Appt time:
Prep For Test:	
Test Results:	

DOCTOR VISITS

Date:	Appt Time:
Physician:	Specialty:
Reason For Visit:	

QUESTIONS/CONCERNS

VITALS

Height:	Weight:
Blood Pressure:	Pulse Rate:
Blood Glucose:	Temperature:

MEDICATION UPDATES

Medication	Dosage	Frequency	Duration

PHYSICIAN DIAGNOSIS / DISCUSSION

TESTS ORDERED

Test/Exam:	Facility
Date:	Appt time:
Prep For Test:	
Test Results:	

Test/Exam:	Facility
Date:	Appt time:
Prep For Test:	
Test Results:	

Test/Exam:	Facility
Date:	Appt time:
Prep For Test:	
Test Results:	

DOCTOR VISITS

Date:	Appt Time:
Physician:	Specialty:
Reason For Visit:	

QUESTIONS/CONCERNS

VITALS

Height:	Weight:
Blood Pressure:	Pulse Rate:
Blood Glucose:	Temperature:

MEDICATION UPDATES

Medication	Dosage	Frequency	Duration

PHYSICIAN DIAGNOSIS / DISCUSSION

TESTS ORDERED

Test/Exam:	Facility
Date:	Appt time:
Prep For Test:	
Test Results:	

Test/Exam:	Facility
Date:	Appt time:
Prep For Test:	
Test Results:	

Test/Exam:	Facility
Date:	Appt time:
Prep For Test:	
Test Results:	

DOCTOR VISITS

Date:	Appt Time:
Physician:	Specialty:
Reason For Visit:	

QUESTIONS/CONCERNS

VITALS

Height:	Weight:
Blood Pressure:	Pulse Rate:
Blood Glucose:	Temperature:

MEDICATION UPDATES

Medication	Dosage	Frequency	Duration

PHYSICIAN DIAGNOSIS / DISCUSSION

TESTS ORDERED

Test/Exam:	Facility
Date:	Appt time:
Prep For Test:	
Test Results:	

Test/Exam:	Facility
Date:	Appt time:
Prep For Test:	
Test Results:	

Test/Exam:	Facility
Date:	Appt time:
Prep For Test:	
Test Results:	

DOCTOR VISITS

Date:	Appt Time:
Physician:	Specialty:
Reason For Visit:	

QUESTIONS/CONCERNS

VITALS

Height:	Weight:
Blood Pressure:	Pulse Rate:
Blood Glucose:	Temperature:

MEDICATION UPDATES

Medication	Dosage	Frequency	Duration

PHYSICIAN DIAGNOSIS / DISCUSSION

TESTS ORDERED

Test/Exam:	Facility
Date:	Appt time:
Prep For Test:	
Test Results:	

Test/Exam:	Facility
Date:	Appt time:
Prep For Test:	
Test Results:	

Test/Exam:	Facility
Date:	Appt time:
Prep For Test:	
Test Results:	

DOCTOR VISITS

Date:	Appt Time:
Physician:	Specialty:
Reason For Visit:	

QUESTIONS/CONCERNS

VITALS

Height:	Weight:
Blood Pressure:	Pulse Rate:
Blood Glucose:	Temperature:

MEDICATION UPDATES

Medication	Dosage	Frequency	Duration

PHYSICIAN DIAGNOSIS / DISCUSSION

TESTS ORDERED

Test/Exam:	Facility
Date:	Appt time:
Prep For Test:	
Test Results:	

Test/Exam:	Facility
Date:	Appt time:
Prep For Test:	
Test Results:	

Test/Exam:	Facility
Date:	Appt time:
Prep For Test:	
Test Results:	

DOCTOR VISITS

Date:	Appt Time:
Physician:	Specialty:
Reason For Visit:	

QUESTIONS/CONCERNS

VITALS

Height:	Weight:
Blood Pressure:	Pulse Rate:
Blood Glucose:	Temperature:

MEDICATION UPDATES

Medication	Dosage	Frequency	Duration

PHYSICIAN DIAGNOSIS / DISCUSSION

TESTS ORDERED

Test/Exam:	Facility
Date:	Appt time:
Prep For Test:	
Test Results:	

Test/Exam:	Facility
Date:	Appt time:
Prep For Test:	
Test Results:	

Test/Exam:	Facility
Date:	Appt time:
Prep For Test:	
Test Results:	

DOCTOR VISITS

Date:	Appt Time:
Physician:	Specialty:
Reason For Visit:	

QUESTIONS/CONCERNS

VITALS

Height:	Weight:
Blood Pressure:	Pulse Rate:
Blood Glucose:	Temperature:

MEDICATION UPDATES

Medication	Dosage	Frequency	Duration

PHYSICIAN DIAGNOSIS / DISCUSSION

TESTS ORDERED

Test/Exam:	Facility
Date:	Appt time:
Prep For Test:	
Test Results:	

Test/Exam:	Facility
Date:	Appt time:
Prep For Test:	
Test Results:	

Test/Exam:	Facility
Date:	Appt time:
Prep For Test:	
Test Results:	

DOCTOR VISITS

Date:	Appt Time:
Physician:	Specialty:
Reason For Visit:	

QUESTIONS/CONCERNS

VITALS

Height:	Weight:
Blood Pressure:	Pulse Rate:
Blood Glucose:	Temperature:

MEDICATION UPDATES

Medication	Dosage	Frequency	Duration

PHYSICIAN DIAGNOSIS / DISCUSSION

TESTS ORDERED

Test/Exam:	Facility
Date:	Appt time:
Prep For Test:	
Test Results:	

Test/Exam:	Facility
Date:	Appt time:
Prep For Test:	
Test Results:	

Test/Exam:	Facility
Date:	Appt time:
Prep For Test:	
Test Results:	

DOCTOR VISITS

Date:	Appt Time:
Physician:	Specialty:
Reason For Visit:	

QUESTIONS/CONCERNS

VITALS

Height:	Weight:
Blood Pressure:	Pulse Rate:
Blood Glucose:	Temperature:

MEDICATION UPDATES

Medication	Dosage	Frequency	Duration

PHYSICIAN DIAGNOSIS / DISCUSSION

TESTS ORDERED

Test/Exam:	Facility
Date:	Appt time:
Prep For Test:	
Test Results:	

Test/Exam:	Facility
Date:	Appt time:
Prep For Test:	
Test Results:	

Test/Exam:	Facility
Date:	Appt time:
Prep For Test:	
Test Results:	

DOCTOR VISITS

Date:	Appt Time:
Physician:	Specialty:
Reason For Visit:	

QUESTIONS/CONCERNS

VITALS

Height:	Weight:
Blood Pressure:	Pulse Rate:
Blood Glucose:	Temperature:

MEDICATION UPDATES

Medication	Dosage	Frequency	Duration

PHYSICIAN DIAGNOSIS / DISCUSSION

TESTS ORDERED

Test/Exam:	Facility
Date:	Appt time:
Prep For Test:	
Test Results:	

Test/Exam:	Facility
Date:	Appt time:
Prep For Test:	
Test Results:	

Test/Exam:	Facility
Date:	Appt time:
Prep For Test:	
Test Results:	

DOCTOR VISITS

Date:	Appt Time:
Physician:	Specialty:
Reason For Visit:	

QUESTIONS/CONCERNS

VITALS

Height:	Weight:
Blood Pressure:	Pulse Rate:
Blood Glucose:	Temperature:

MEDICATION UPDATES

Medication	Dosage	Frequency	Duration

PHYSICIAN DIAGNOSIS / DISCUSSION

TESTS ORDERED

Test/Exam:	Facility
Date:	Appt time:
Prep For Test:	
Test Results:	

Test/Exam:	Facility
Date:	Appt time:
Prep For Test:	
Test Results:	

Test/Exam:	Facility
Date:	Appt time:
Prep For Test:	
Test Results:	

DOCTOR VISITS

Date:	Appt Time:
Physician:	Specialty:
Reason For Visit:	

QUESTIONS/CONCERNS

VITALS

Height:	Weight:
Blood Pressure:	Pulse Rate:
Blood Glucose:	Temperature:

MEDICATION UPDATES

Medication	Dosage	Frequency	Duration

PHYSICIAN DIAGNOSIS / DISCUSSION

TESTS ORDERED

Test/Exam:	Facility
Date:	Appt time:
Prep For Test:	
Test Results:	

Test/Exam:	Facility
Date:	Appt time:
Prep For Test:	
Test Results:	

Test/Exam:	Facility
Date:	Appt time:
Prep For Test:	
Test Results:	

DOCTOR VISITS

Date:	Appt Time:
Physician:	Specialty:
Reason For Visit:	

QUESTIONS/CONCERNS

VITALS

Height:	Weight:
Blood Pressure:	Pulse Rate:
Blood Glucose:	Temperature:

MEDICATION UPDATES

Medication	Dosage	Frequency	Duration

PHYSICIAN DIAGNOSIS / DISCUSSION

TESTS ORDERED

Test/Exam:	Facility
Date:	Appt time:
Prep For Test:	
Test Results:	

Test/Exam:	Facility
Date:	Appt time:
Prep For Test:	
Test Results:	

Test/Exam:	Facility
Date:	Appt time:
Prep For Test:	
Test Results:	

DOCTOR VISITS

Date:	Appt Time:
Physician:	Specialty:
Reason For Visit:	

QUESTIONS/CONCERNS

VITALS

Height:	Weight:
Blood Pressure:	Pulse Rate:
Blood Glucose:	Temperature:

MEDICATION UPDATES

Medication	Dosage	Frequency	Duration

PHYSICIAN DIAGNOSIS / DISCUSSION

TESTS ORDERED

Test/Exam:	Facility
Date:	Appt time:
Prep For Test:	
Test Results:	

Test/Exam:	Facility
Date:	Appt time:
Prep For Test:	
Test Results:	

Test/Exam:	Facility
Date:	Appt time:
Prep For Test:	
Test Results:	

DOCTOR VISITS

Date:	Appt Time:
Physician:	Specialty:
Reason For Visit:	

QUESTIONS/CONCERNS

VITALS

Height:	Weight:
Blood Pressure:	Pulse Rate:
Blood Glucose:	Temperature:

MEDICATION UPDATES

Medication	Dosage	Frequency	Duration

PHYSICIAN DIAGNOSIS / DISCUSSION

TESTS ORDERED

Test/Exam:	Facility
Date:	Appt time:
Prep For Test:	
Test Results:	

Test/Exam:	Facility
Date:	Appt time:
Prep For Test:	
Test Results:	

Test/Exam:	Facility
Date:	Appt time:
Prep For Test:	
Test Results:	

DOCTOR VISITS

Date:	Appt Time:
Physician:	Specialty:
Reason For Visit:	

QUESTIONS/CONCERNS

VITALS

Height:	Weight:
Blood Pressure:	Pulse Rate:
Blood Glucose:	Temperature:

MEDICATION UPDATES

Medication	Dosage	Frequency	Duration

PHYSICIAN DIAGNOSIS / DISCUSSION

TESTS ORDERED

Test/Exam:	Facility
Date:	Appt time:
Prep For Test:	
Test Results:	

Test/Exam:	Facility
Date:	Appt time:
Prep For Test:	
Test Results:	

Test/Exam:	Facility
Date:	Appt time:
Prep For Test:	
Test Results:	

NOTES

WALLET SIZED MEDICATION/VITAMEN/SUPPLEMENT CARDS
CUT ON THE OUTER MARGIN/FOLD ON THE CENTER MARGIN

Name:		MEDICATION	DOSAGE
Address:			
Phone:			
MEDICATION	**DOSAGE**		

Name:		MEDICATION	DOSAGE
Address:			
Phone:			
MEDICATION	**DOSAGE**		

WALLET SIZED MEDICATION/VITAMEN/SUPPLEMENT CARDS
CUT ON THE OUTER MARGIN/FOLD ON THE CENTER MARGIN

Name:		MEDICATION	DOSAGE
Address:			
Phone:			
MEDICATION	DOSAGE		

Name:		MEDICATION	DOSAGE
Address:			
Phone:			
MEDICATION	DOSAGE		

WALLET SIZED EMERGENCY INFORMATION CARDS
CUT ON THE OUTER MARGIN/FOLD ON THE CENTER MARGIN

Name:	BLOOD TYPE	
Address:	DONOR	YES/NO
Phone:	RESUSITATE	YES/NO
EMERGENCY CONTACTS/DOCTORS	HIGH BLOOD PRESSURE	YES/NO
Name:	DIABETES (INSULIN/ORAL)	**YES/NO**
Phone:	PACEMAKER	YES/NO
Name:	MEDICATONS	DOSE
Phone:		
Physician:		
Phone:		
Physician:		
Phone:		

Name:	BLOOD TYPE	
Address:	DONOR	YES/NO
Phone:	RESUSITATE	YES/NO
EMERGENCY CONTACTS/DOCTORS	HIGH BLOOD PRESSURE	YES/NO
Name:	DIABETES (INSULIN/ORAL)	**YES/NO**
Phone:	PACEMAKER	YES/NO
Name:	MEDICATONS	DOSE
Phone:		
Physician:		
Phone:		
Physician:		
Phone:		

WALLET SIZED EMERGENCY INFORMATION CARDS
CUT ON THE OUTER MARGIN/FOLD ON THE CENTER MARGIN

Name:	BLOOD TYPE	
Address:	DONOR	YES/NO
Phone:	RESUSITATE	YES/NO
EMERGENCY CONTACTS/DOCTORS	HIGH BLOOD PRESSURE	YES/NO
Name:	DIABETES (INSULIN/ORAL)	**YES/NO**
Phone:	PACEMAKER	YES/NO
Name:	MEDICATONS	DOSE
Phone:		
Physician:		
Phone:		
Physician:		
Phone:		

Name:	BLOOD TYPE	
Address:	DONOR	YES/NO
Phone:	RESUSITATE	YES/NO
EMERGENCY CONTACTS/DOCTORS	HIGH BLOOD PRESSURE	YES/NO
Name:	DIABETES (INSULIN/ORAL)	**YES/NO**
Phone:	PACEMAKER	YES/NO
Name:	MEDICATONS	DOSE
Phone:		
Physician:		
Phone:		
Physician:		
Phone:		

Made in the USA
Monee, IL
11 January 2022